THE HEALTHY GOUT DIET RECIPES FOR BEGINNERS 2024

Simple and Delicious Low-Purine Meal Guide for Promoting Balanced Wellness

By

Milla Chase

Copyright © 2024 by Milla Chase

Table of content

Introduction

Managing your diet might be particularly difficult when you have gout. You may have felt the stress of trying to figure out what you can and cannot eat, the irritation of flare-ups, and the pain that interferes with your everyday life. The good news? You're not alone. The similar path is being followed by thousands of individuals who are learning how to avoid items that make them uncomfortable while maintaining a healthy nutritional balance. The even better news? The purpose of this book is to ease your trip.

Not just another cookbook, *The Healthy Gout Diet Recipes for Beginners 2024* is your mentor, your friend, and your source of support. It was designed to help you take back control, enjoy food, and live your life without worrying about the next flare-up all the time. You should consume food that makes you feel your best, tastes amazing, and nourishes you. That's precisely what this book does.

You will find yourself in a universe where food is used as a healing instrument rather than a cause of anxiety as soon as you access these pages. You will be exposed to dishes that satisfy your dietary requirements while also being tasty, simple to prepare, and sufficiently diverse to keep your taste buds engaged. Bid farewell to monotonous, repetitive meals and welcome to tasty choices that complement your way of life. With basic ingredients that are readily available in any grocery shop, each recipe has been thoughtfully created to be beginner-friendly. Simple, effective cooking without any daunting instructions or intricate methods.

What makes this so crucial? Because the most effective way to manage gout may be to consume the proper meals. You may prevent painful episodes, decrease uric acid levels, and lessen inflammation by eating foods that are good for your health. It's a step toward leading a more lively and self-assured life in addition to a healthy one. Imagine having meals you look forward to, waking up pain-free, and knowing you're actively working to improve your health.

The purpose of this book is to simplify your life. You'll discover a range of meals that won't hinder your development, including filling breakfasts, stimulating lunches, gratifying dinners, and even snacks and sweets. To help you enjoy your creations, each recipe includes precise preparation timings, serving suggestions, and easy-to-follow directions. Who wouldn't like a little sweetness or a savoury delight without feeling guilty or running the danger of a flare-up, let's face it? We've taken care to provide choices that also satiate those desires.

It might be intimidating to start a new diet, particularly if it's for health reasons. You may be thinking about the following queries at the moment: "Will I really enjoy these meals at all ?" "Are the ingredients in my area?" "Will the effort be worthwhile?" Yes, yes, and certainly is the response. All of these recipes have been created to be fun, useful, and efficient. You'll discover that a well planned diet may be surprisingly tasty. These are recipes you'll be thrilled to serve and enjoy, not meals you'll have to make yourself eat.

One dish at a time, you're managing your health rather than simply cooking. You're embracing change, supporting your body, and discovering new ways to enjoy food with every meal you cook. Start your path to a more pain-free, balanced existence with this book. So get your hands dirty, get to the kitchen, and prepare to discover a world of gout-friendly, healthful meals that will motivate you and change the way you eat.

Here to empower you is ***The Healthy Gout Diet Recipes for Beginners 2024*** . Accept it, use it in your cooking, and most all, savour each taste.

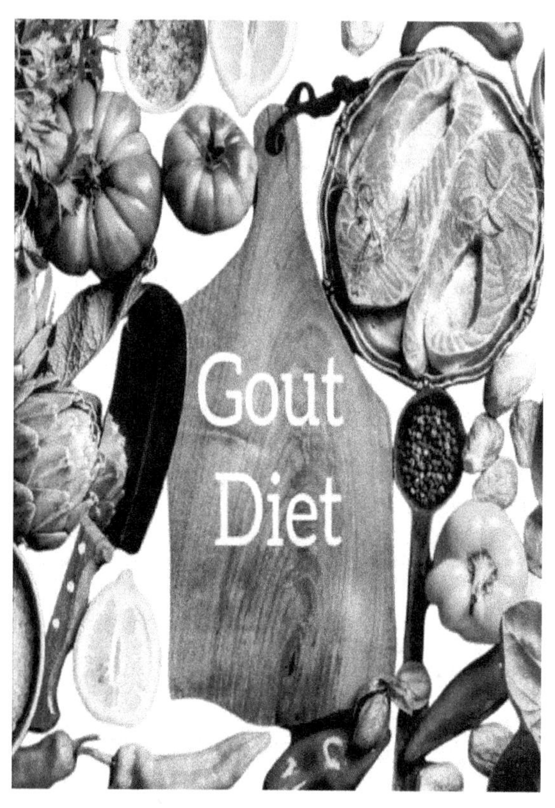

Gout
Diet

Chapter 1: Understanding Gout

What is Gout?

Gout, a kind of arthritis, is characterised by abrupt, intense joint pain, edema, and redness. The big toe is the joint most often affected, although it may also happen in the ankles, knees, wrists, and fingers. When blood uric acid levels are excessive, gout develops. Normally, uric acid is created when your body breaks down chemicals called purines, which are included in certain diets. Urine is often the body's method of eliminating uric acid.

However, your body begins to generate sharp, needle-like crystals in your joints if there is an excess of uric acid or if it is unable to eliminate it effectively. Gout attacks are brought on by the excruciating inflammation that these crystals produce.

Gout flares up without warning and often wakes you up in the middle of the night with excruciating agony. The afflicted joint may be very sensitive to the touch, heated, and swollen. The proper care and lifestyle modifications, including modifying your diet to reduce uric acid levels, may help manage gout. Gout may be effectively managed by avoiding purine-rich meals, drinking enough water, and keeping a healthy weight.

Hyperuricemia, or elevated uric acid levels in the body, is the cause of gout. Purines, which are naturally occurring compounds in your body and in certain meals, are broken down by your body to produce uric acid, a waste product. The key to understanding why gout occurs is knowing how uric acid and purines function in your body.

Uric Acid and Purine Metabolism

Purines are chemical substances that are present in many meals, particularly meat, shellfish, and alcohol, and that are also a component of your body's DNA. Uric acid is a result of the breakdown of purines in your body. Normally, your blood dissolves this uric acid, which is then processed by your kidneys and expelled from your body via urine.

However, uric acid accumulates in your blood if your body creates too much of it or if your kidneys are unable to eliminate it enough. Inflammation, discomfort, and swelling may result from the excess uric acid forming small, pointed crystals in your joints and tissues. The primary cause of people's excruciating gout episodes is these uric acid crystals.

Gout may result from elevated uric acid levels for a number of causes. These variables fall into two groups: *those that raise the formation of uric acid and those that lower its elimination.*

Increased Production of Uric Acid

- **Diet High in Purines**: Consuming purine-rich meals might cause uric acid levels to rise. Purines are found in high concentrations in foods such as red meat, organ meats (liver, kidneys), seafood, and alcohol (particularly beer). These foods raise your chance of developing gout because they cause your body to create more uric acid.
- **Obesity:** Uric acid levels are more likely to be increased in those who are overweight or obese. This is due to the fact that being overweight increases the body's production of uric acid and decreases its capacity to remove it.
- **Some Medical Conditions**: Diabetes, hypertension, and metabolic syndrome are among the illnesses that may cause an increase in uric acid production. These illnesses have an impact on how the body processes uric acid and may

make it more difficult for your kidneys to remove it.

- **Kidney Function**: The removal of uric acid from your body is mostly the responsibility of your kidneys. Your blood may accumulate uric acid if your kidneys aren't functioning properly because they may not be able to filter it out completely. For instance, gout is more common in those with chronic renal illness.
- **Dehydration**: Your body has less fluid to assist eliminate uric acid via urine when you're dehydrated. Uric acid levels may increase as a result, increasing the possibility of joint crystal formation.
- **Some medications**: Certain drugs may affect the way your body gets rid of uric acid. For instance, diuretics, which are often recommended to treat high blood pressure, might cause your body to retain less water and make it more difficult for your kidneys to eliminate uric acid.

Additional Gout Risk Factors

Gout may be caused by a number of other variables outside food and renal function, including:

1.   **Genetic:** Gout may run in families, Because some individuals naturally make more uric acid or have a harder time removing it, you may be at a higher risk of developing gout if you have a family history of it.
2.   **Gender and Age:** Men are more likely than women to have gout, particularly in middle age. But women's uric acid levels rise after menopause, increasing their chance of getting gout later in life.
3.   **Drinking Alcohol:** Because it increases the formation of uric acid and decreases its removal, drinking alcohol, particularly beer and liquor, may raise uric acid levels.

High uric acid levels in the body, which may be brought on by either an excess of uric acid being produced or the body's incapacity to properly remove it, are the cause of gout.

Common Symptoms of gout

Usually, gout results in abrupt, severe joint pain in one or more joints. Although it may affect the ankles, knees, elbows, wrists, and fingers, the big toe is the joint most often impacted. You may wake up in excruciating agony from a gout attack, which often happens at night. In addition to discomfort, the afflicted joint may be swollen, red, and very sensitive to touch. The joint's surrounding skin may feel heated or glossy. If treatment is not received, the frequency of these flare-ups may increase over time and may last anywhere from a few days to weeks.

Importance of Early Management

Gout must be treated early to avoid causing long-term joint damage. Gout may cause more frequent and severe flare-ups, which can cause irreversible damage to the afflicted joints, if treatment is not received. In addition to causing kidney stones, uric acid crystals may accumulate under the skin over time and form lumps known as tophi. Uric acid levels may be lowered, symptoms can be managed, and more episodes can be avoided with early therapy that includes medication and dietary modifications. You can preserve your joints and enhance your general quality of life by treating gout early.

Chapter 2: The Role of Diet in Gout Management

The Impact of Diet on Uric Acid Levels

Because diet has a direct impact on your body's uric acid levels, it is important for controlling gout. Purines, which are naturally occurring compounds in many foods and your body, are broken down by your body to form uric acid. The excruciating inflammation linked to gout may be brought on by crystals forming in your joints as a result of high uric acid levels.

High-Purine Foods to Avoid

Purine-rich foods should be avoided or consumed in moderation for treating gout. These meals may raise your body's uric acid production, which raises the possibility of excruciating flare-ups of gout. Key high-purine meals to stay away from include:

- **Red Meat:** Red meats such as beef, lamb, and hog are high in purines. Gout attacks may result from eating these foods because they increase uric acid levels.

- **Organ meats**: Meats from the liver, kidneys, and other organs are particularly rich in purines and should be avoided since they may cause a substantial increase in uric acid.

- **The seafood**: Due to their high purine content, certain seafood—including sardines, anchovies, herring, mackerel, scallops, and shellfish (shrimp, lobster)—can aggravate gout.

- **Alcohol:** Alcoholic drinks, particularly those containing yeast, such as beer and liquor, may raise uric acid levels. Alcohol poses a dual hazard as it impairs the body's capacity to flush out uric acid.

- **Sugar-filled foods and beverages**: Despite not having a lot of purines, meals rich in fructose, sweetened juices, and sodas may boost uric acid levels. They should be avoided.

Varieties of purine-free meals may help control gout by lowering uric acid levels. You may include these items in your diet without restriction if you have gout:

- **The fruits and vegetables**: Gout may benefit from most fruits and vegetables since they are low in purines. Particularly beneficial are citrus fruits, apples, strawberries, and cherries. Kale, spinach, and broccoli are other excellent vegetables.

- **Whole grains:** Whole wheat, quinoa, brown rice, and oats are among the foods that are low in purines and provide vital nutrients. In addition to lowering uric acid levels, these grains support general health.

- **Dairy Products Low in Fat:** Low-fat cheeses, milk, and yoghurt may lower uric acid levels in addition to being low in purines. One effective strategy to control gout is to include them into your diet.

- **Nuts and Seeds:** Nuts and seeds that are low in purines, such as walnuts, flaxseeds, chia seeds, and almonds, may provide minerals and healthful fats without increasing uric acid levels.

- **Plant-based proteins and eggs**: Eggs are a rich source of protein and low in purines. A few more great plant-based protein sources include tofu, beans, and lentils.

- **Water**: Hydration is essential for gout management. By assisting the kidneys in eliminating uric acid, drinking plenty of water lowers the chance of crystal formation.

Avoiding foods rich in purines and choosing meals low in purines can help you manage your gout and lessen the frequency of excruciating flare-ups. These dietary adjustments may significantly improve your health and well-being.

Chapter 3: Delicious Recipes for Gout Management

Breakfast Recipes

Fresh Berries with Oatmeal

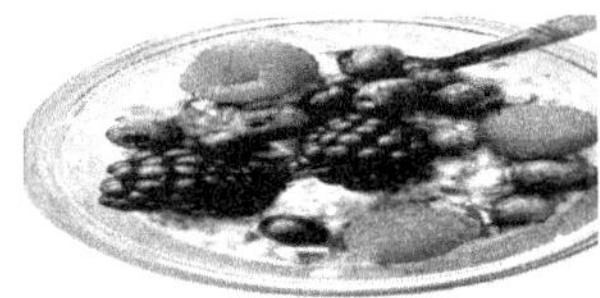

Ingredients:

-One cup of rolled oats
-Two cups of low-fat milk or water
-One cup of fresh berry mixture (raspberries, blueberries, and strawberries)
-One teaspoon of cinnamon

Preparation Procedures:

1. Bring milk or water to a boil in a saucepan.
2. Turn down the heat to low and stir in the rolled oats.
3. Cook, stirring periodically, for 5 minutes.
4. Turn off the heat and add the cinnamon.
5. Before serving, sprinkle mixed berries on top.

Duration : 10 minutes.

Serving Method: Transfer to a bowl and serve warm.

Nutritional values: Calories: 300, Protein: 10g, Carbs: 45g, Fats: 8g and Fibre: 8g

Parfait with Greek Yoghourt

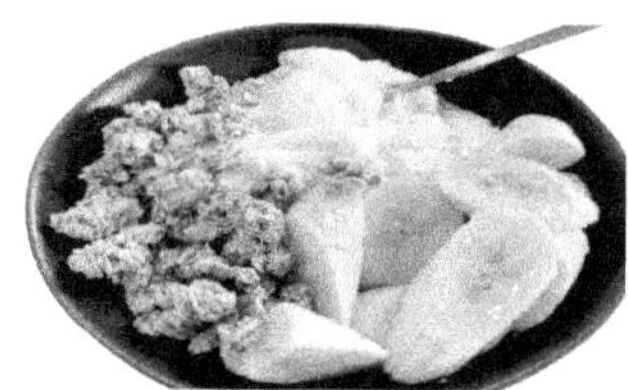

Ingredients:

-One cup of Greek yoghourt
-One medium banana, cut into slices Half a cup of granola

Preparation Procedures:

1. Place half of the Greek yoghurt in a glass or dish.
2. Top the yoghurt with half of the banana slices.
3. Cover the banana with half of the granola.
4. Continue layering the remaining granola, banana, and yoghurt.
5. Serve right away.

Duration : 5 minutes.
Serving Method: Pour into a bowl or glass.

Nutritional values: Calories:~455, Protein: 18 g, Fat: 7 g, Carbohydrates: 82 g, Fibre: 7 g

Avocado Toast

- One ripe avocado
- A pair of wholegrain bread slices
- One teaspoon of lemon juice
- Salt and pepper.

1. Before it becomes golden brown, toast the wholegrain bread.
2. Mash the avocado, lemon juice, salt, and pepper in a bowl.
3. Evenly cover each piece of bread with mashed avocado.
4. Optional: Add sliced radishes or tomatoes on top.
5. Serve right away.

:10 minutes.

: serve in a plate

Nutritional values: Calories: 250, Protein: 6g, Carbs: 24g, Fats: 15g, Fibre: 7g

Spinach and Scrambled Eggs

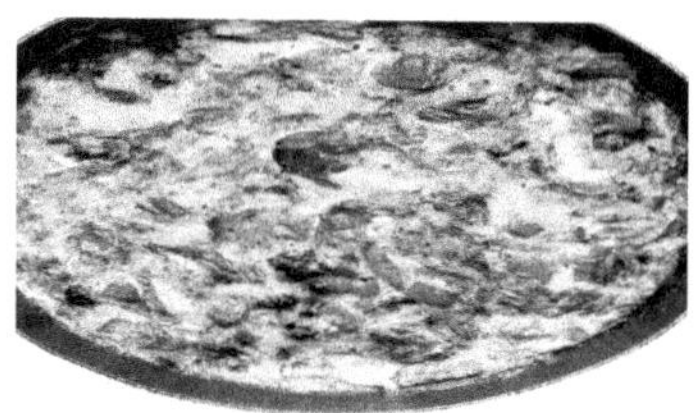

Ingredients:

-Two huge eggs
-One cup of freshly chopped spinach
-One teaspoon of olive oil
-Salt and pepper.

Preparation Procedures:

1. Whisk the eggs, salt, and pepper in a bowl.
2. In a non-stick skillet, heat the olive oil over medium heat.
3. Cook the chopped spinach until it wilts.
4. Gently whisk the eggs after pouring them into the skillet.
5. Cook for 3–4 minutes, or until the eggs are just set.

Duration : 10 minutes.
Serving Method: Warm food should be served on a dish.

Nutritional values: Calories:~187, Protein:12 g, Fat: 14 g, Carbohydrates: 2 g
Fibre: 0.7 g

Banana and kale smoothie

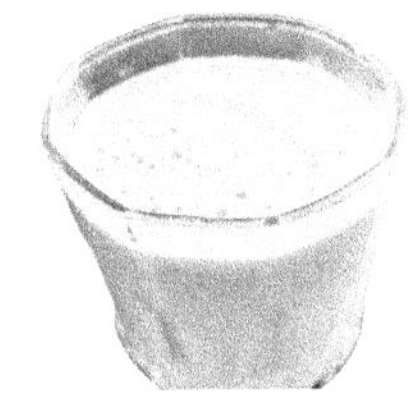

Ingredients:

-One cup of chopped kale

-One medium banana

-A quarter cup of low-fat yoghurts

-One cup of almond milk

Preparation Procedures:

1. Put the kale, banana, yoghurt, and almond milk in a blender.
2. Blend until smooth at high speed.
3. To get the right consistency, add more almond milk if it's too thick.
4. If necessary, taste and adjust sweetness.
5. Transfer to a glass and serve right away.

Duration : 5 minutes.

Serving Method : it in a glass.

Nutritional values: ~Calories: 203, Protein: 6 g Fat: 4 g, Carbohydrates: 36 g, Fibre: 5 g

Chia Seed Pudding

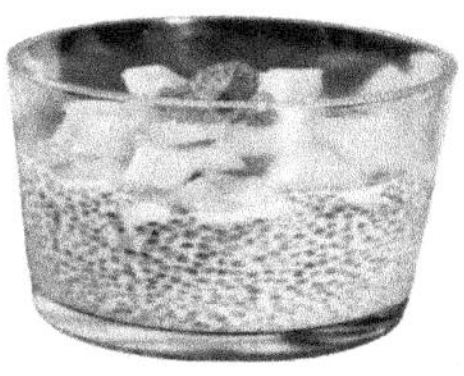

Ingredients:

-Half a cup of chia seeds

-One cup of almond milk

-One spoonful of maple syrup or honey

- Fresh fruit to garnish

Preparation Procedures:

1. Combine the honey, almond milk, and chia seeds in a dish.
2. Give it a good stir and let it for five minutes.
3. To avoid clumping, stir one more.
4. Cover and chill overnight or for at least two hours.
5. Before serving, sprinkle some fresh fruit on top.

Duration: 2 hours (5 minutes for preparation)

Serving method: Serve cold in a jar or dish.

Nutritional values: Calories: ~360, Protein: 10 g, Fat: 20 g, Carbohydrates: 45 g, Fibre: 18 g

Lunch Recipes

Quinoa salad with Vegetables

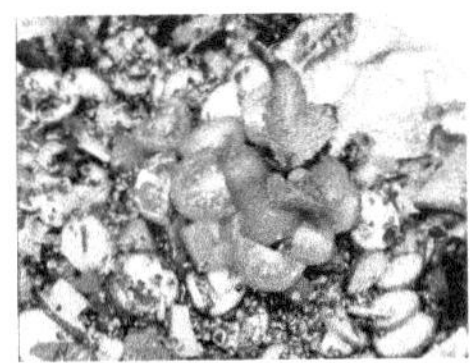

Ingredients:

-A cup of cooked quinoa

-half a cup of sliced cucumber

-half a cup of cherry tomatoes, cut in half, - one tablespoon of olive oil

 - Salt and pepper

 - handful of parsley chopped (Optional)

 - handful of mint leaves (Optional)

Preparation procedures:

1. Put the cooked quinoa, cherry tomatoes, and cucumber in a big bowl.

2. Add salt and pepper to taste and drizzle with olive oil.

3. Gently toss to mix all items together.

4. Give it five minutes to settle so the flavours can combine.

5. You may serve it cold or at room temperature.

Duration: 10 minutes

Serving method: served in a bowl

Nutritional values: Calories: ~270, Protein: 8g, Carbs: 40g, Fats: 9g, Fibre: 7g

Turkey Wrap

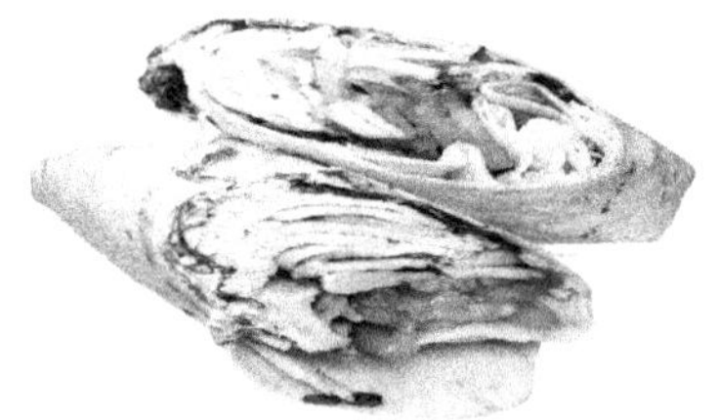

Ingredients:

- one 4-ounce portion of sliced turkey breast
- 1 whole-grain tortilla
- ½ sliced of avocado
- 1 cup of Shredded lettuce

Preparation procedures:

1. Place the tortilla on a clean surface.
2. Top with lettuce, avocado, and turkey slices.
3. Tuck the edges of the tortilla in as you securely roll it.
4. Cut the wrap in two pieces.
5. You may package for later or serve right now.

Duration: **5** minutes
Serving method: **A plate is the ideal serving vessel.**

Nutritional values: Calories: ~375, Protein: 28 g, Fat: 22 g, Carbohydrates: 30 g, Fibre: 12 g

Lentils soup

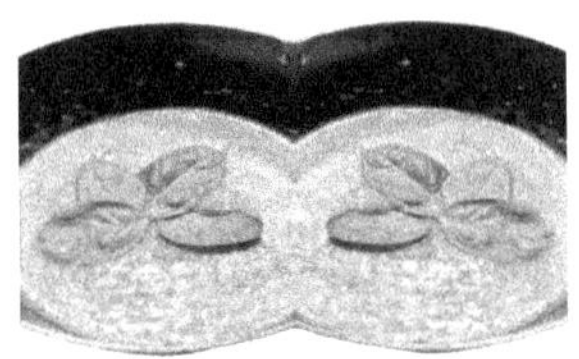

Ingredients:

- One cup of rinsed and drained dry lentils; - one medium onion
- two diced carrots
- two diced celery stalks
- two minced garlic cloves
- One teaspoon of olive oil
- One teaspoon of ground turmeric (Optional)
- Six cups of low-sodium vegetable broth (freshly cut parsley for decoration)
- Salt and pepper

Preparation procedures:

1. Heat olive oil in a big saucepan over medium heat. Add the chopped celery, carrots, and onion. Sauté until they are tender, approximately 5 minutes.

2. Add the turmeric (if using) and minced garlic, and simmer for one more minute until aromatic.

3. Add the lentils and vegetable broth. Once they are added, bring the mixture to a boil.

4. Lower the heat to low, cover the saucepan, and simmer until the veggies and lentils are soft, 25 to 30 minutes.

5. Season with salt and pepper. Fill dishes with the soup and sprinkle with fresh parsley.

Duration : **40 minutes**

Nutritional value: calories : ~180, Protein :12g, carbohydrates: 28g, fibre:12g, and fat:2g

Hummus and Veggie

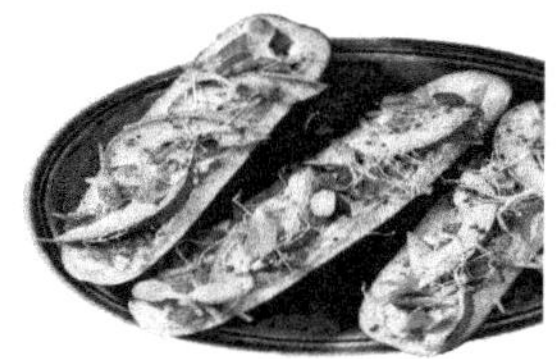

Ingredients:

- 1 cup hummus
- 1 cup carrot sticks
- One cup of cucumber slices
- Avocado (Optional)

- An whole cup of bell pepper strips

1. On a dish, arrange the bell pepper strips, cucumber slices, and carrot sticks.
2. Put a little dish of hummus in the middle.
3. Present a tray of fresh veggies beside.
4. Savour them while dipping.
5. Keep leftovers refrigerated.

Duration: 5 minutes
Serving method: serve by placing it on a dish.

Nutritional value: Calories: ~200, Protein: 6g, Carbs: 25g, Fats: 9g, Fibre: 7g

Tuna salad

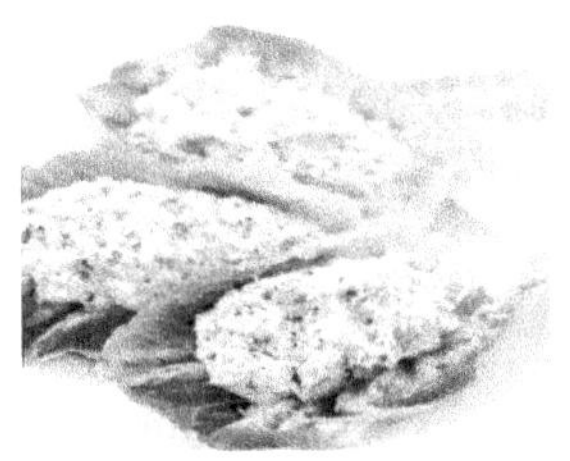

Ingredients:

- 1 can (5 oz) of drained tuna in water
- One-sixth cup Greek yoghourt
- One sliced celery stalk

- one teaspoon of lemon juice
- Salt and pepper
- onions (Optional)

1. Put the lemon juice, celery, Greek yoghurt, and drained tuna in a bowl.
2. Add salt and pepper to taste and mix well.
3. Present on a bed of lettuce or on whole-grain toast.
4. If preferred, chill for ten minutes in the refrigerator.
5. Present right away.

Duration: 10 minutes
Serving method: Put on a sandwich or platter.

Nutritional values: Calories: ~157 , Protein: 26g, Fat: 3g, Carbohydrates: 4g Fibre: 1 g

Cottage Cheese with Pineapple

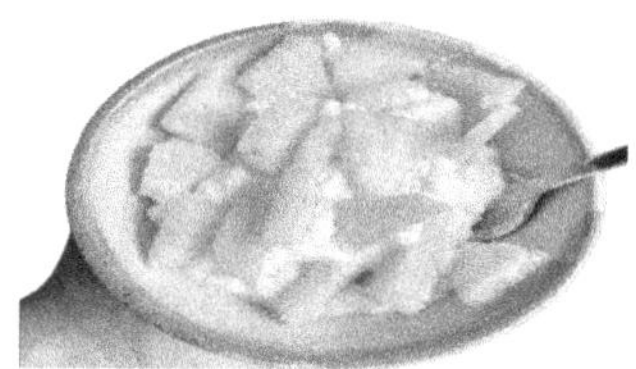

Ingredients:

- 1 cup cottage cheese
- ½ cup pieces of fresh pineapple

1. Place the Spoon cottage cheese inside a bowl.
2. Place fresh pineapple slices on top.
3. Gently stir to mix.
4. For a cool snack, serve right away or refrigerate.
5. Savour as a snack or small lunch.

Duration: 5 minutes
Serving method: This dish should be served in a bowl.

Nutritional values: Calories:~ 200, Protein: 14 g, Carbohydrates: 28 g, Fibre: 1 gram, Fat: 3 grams

Dinner Recipes

Grilled Chicken with Steamed Broccoli

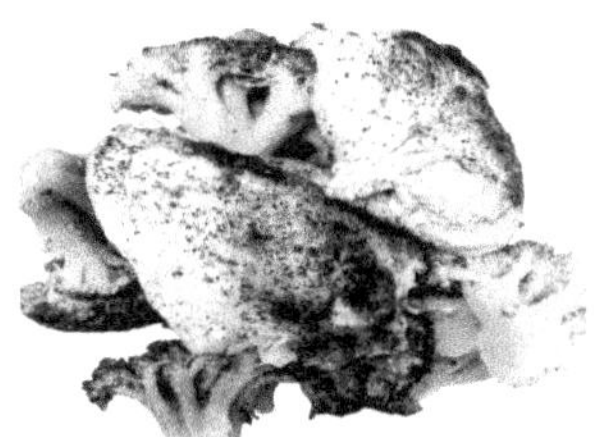

Ingredients:

- 2 boneless, skinless chicken breasts
- Two cups of florets of broccoli
- One tablespoon of olive oil
- Salt and pepper

1. Set the grill's temperature to medium-high.
2. Season chicken breasts with salt and pepper after brushing them with olive oil.
3. The chicken should be cooked through after grilling for 6–7 minutes on each side.
4. In a saucepan, steam broccoli until it is tender, approximately 5 minutes.
5. Serve steamed broccoli with grilled chicken.

Duration: 20 minutes.
Serving method: The recommended method of serving is to use a plate.

Nutritional values: Calories: ~280, Protein: 25g, Carbs: 12g, Fats: 10g, Fibre: 5g

Mixed Vegetables with Stir-Fried Tofu

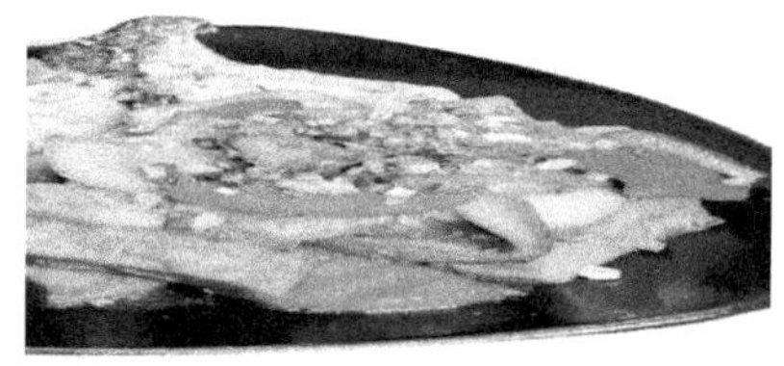

Ingredients:

-14 ounces of diced firm tofu
- Two cups of mixed veggies (carrots, broccoli, and bell peppers)
 - One tablespoon of olive oil
 - Two teaspoons of soy sauce with reduced sodium
 - Salt and pepper.

1. In a big skillet, heat the olive oil over medium-high heat.
2. Stir-fry the cubed tofu for 5–6 minutes, or until it becomes golden brown.
3. Stir-fry the mixed veggies for a further three to four minutes, or until they are crisp-tender.
 4. Stir well after adding the soy sauce and seasoning with salt and pepper.
 5. Serve hot on its own or over brown rice.

15 minutes.
Transfer to a bowl.

Nutritional values: Calories: ~220, Protein: 12g, Carbs: 18g, Fats: 10g, Fibre: 6g

Baked Salmon with Asparagus

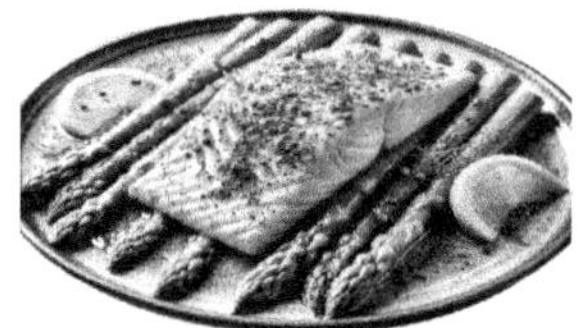

Ingredients :

-2 salmon fillets (4 oz each)
- One bunch of cut asparagus
- One tablespoon of olive oil
- Lemon wedge
- Salt and pepper

Preparation Procedures:

1. Set the oven temperature to 375°F (190°C).
2. Place asparagus and salmon fillets on a baking sheet.
3. Season with salt and pepper and drizzle each with olive oil.
4. The salmon should flake easily with a fork after 15 minutes of baking.
5. Accompany with slices of lemon.

Time: **20 minutes**
Serving Method: **Present on a platter.**

Nutritional values: Calories: ~300, Protein: 22g, Carbs: 8g, Fats: 20g, Fibre: 4g

Zucchini Noodles with Marinara Sauce

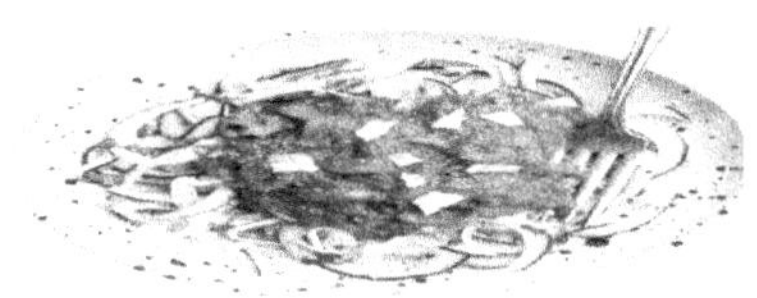

Ingredients:

- 2 medium zucchini, spiralized
- One cup of marinara sauce with reduced sodium
- One teaspoon of Italian spice and one tablespoon of olive oil
- Parmesan cheese, grated (optional)

Preparation Procedures:

1. In a pan, heat the olive oil over medium heat.
2. Sauté the spiralized zucchini for two to three minutes, or until it becomes somewhat tender.
3. Cook for a further three to four minutes after adding the marinara sauce and Italian spice.
4. If preferred, sprinkle with grated Parmesan and serve hot.
5. Savour right now.

Duration : 10 minutes.
Serving method: Transfer to a bowl.

Nutritional values: Calories: ~150, Protein: 5g, Carbs: 20g, Fats: 6g, Fibre: 6g

Black Bean Tacos

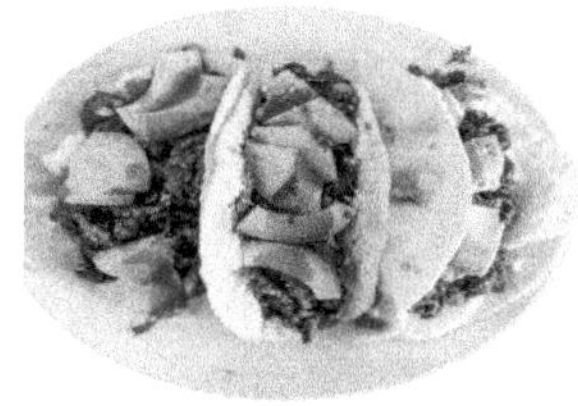

Ingredients:

- 1 can (15 oz) of rinsed and drained black beans
-Four corn tortillas
- One sliced avocado and half a cup of salsa
- Garnish with fresh cilantro (optional)

Preparation Procedures:

1. Heat the black beans in a small saucepan over medium heat until they are well heated.
2. In a pan, warm the corn tortillas for about 30 seconds on each side.
3. Put the tacos together by stuffing each tortilla with salsa, avocado slices, and black beans.
4. If preferred, garnish with fresh cilantro.
5. Serve right away.

Duration: 10 minutes.
Serving method : serve on a plate.

Nutritional values: Calories: ~250, Protein: 10g, Carbs: 35g, Fats: 8g, Fibre: 10g

Vegetable Fried Rice

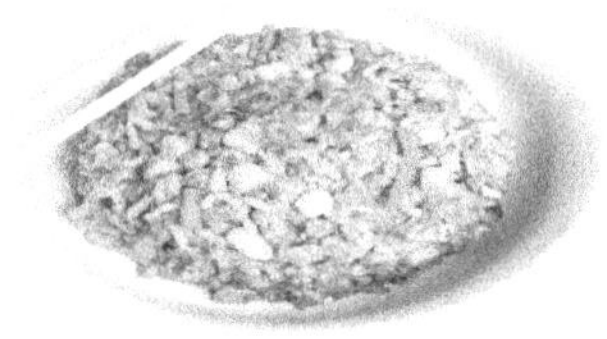

Ingredients :

- 2 cups cooked brown rice
- 1 cup mixed veggies (peas, carrots, and corn)
- 2 eggs, softly beaten
-Soy sauce, one tablespoon
- One tablespoon of olive oil

Preparation Procedures:

1. Heat the olive oil over medium heat in a pan.
2. Sauté the mixed veggies for two to three minutes.
3. After pushing the veggies aside, add the beaten eggs and scramble them until they are done.
4. Mix well after adding the cooked rice and soy sauce.

5. Cook for a further two to three minutes, or until well cooked.

Duration : 15 minutes.
Serving method :In a bowl, serve hot.

Nutritional values: Calories: ~230, Protein: 7g, Carbs: 38g, Fats: 5g, Fibre: 4g

Snacks

Apple Slices with Almond Butter

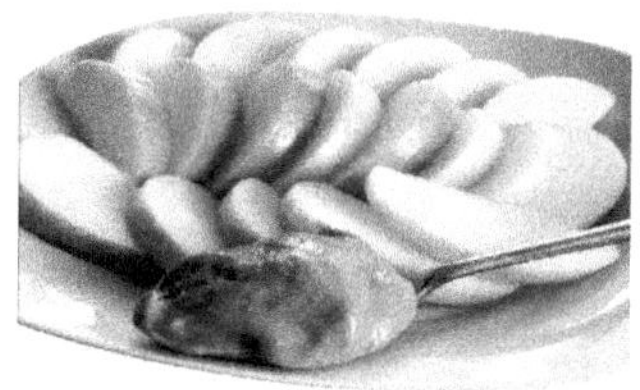

Ingredients:

-two tablespoons of almond butter
- one slice of medium apple

Preparation procedures:

1. Slice the apple into wedges after washing it.
2. Transfer almond butter into a little bowl.

3. Drizzle almond butter over apple slices.

4. Savour as a nutritious appetiser.

5. Refrigerate any remaining almond butter.

Duration: 5 minutes

Serving method: *It* is served on a platter.

Nutritional values: Calories: ~150, Protein: 3g, Carbs: 20g, Fats: 6g, Fibre: 4g

Carrot Sticks with Hummus

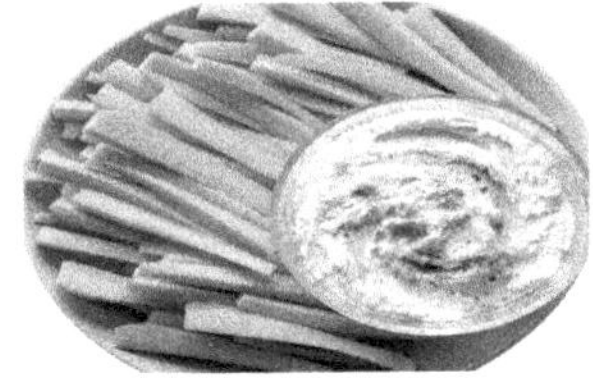

Ingredients:

- 2 big carrots, sliced into sticks
- ½ cup hummus

Preparation procedures:

1. Slice the carrots into sticks after peeling.

2. Transfer the hummus to a little bowl.

3. Present carrot sticks with hummus on the side.

4. Savour as a crispy delicacy.

5. Refrigerate any remaining hummus.

Duration: **5 minutes**
Serving method: **In order to serve, place it on a dish.**

Nutritional values: **Calories: ~130, Protein: 4g, Carbs: 15g, Fats: 6g, Fibre: 5g**

Rice Cakes with Avocado

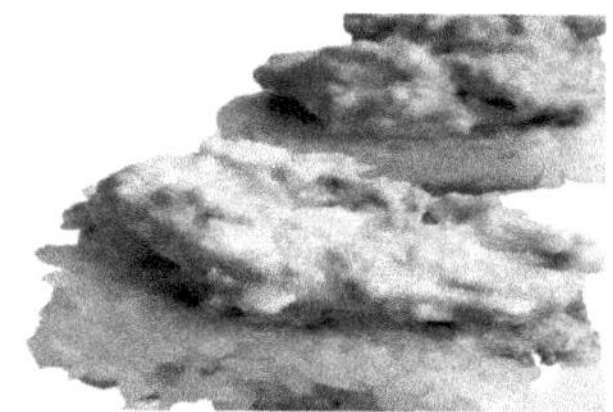

Ingredients:

- 2 rice cakes
- ½ ripe Smashed avocado
- salt and pepper to taste

Preparation procedures:

1. Add salt and pepper to a bowl and mash the avocado.
2. Top each rice cake with an equal layer of mashed avocado.
3. Adding sliced tomatoes or radishes on top is optional.
4. Present right away.
5. Refrigerate any avocado that is left over.

Duration: **5 minutes**

 A plate is the ideal serving vessel.

 Calories: ~170, Protein: 3g, Carbs: 22g, Fats: 8g, Fibre: 4g

Popcorn (Air-Popped)

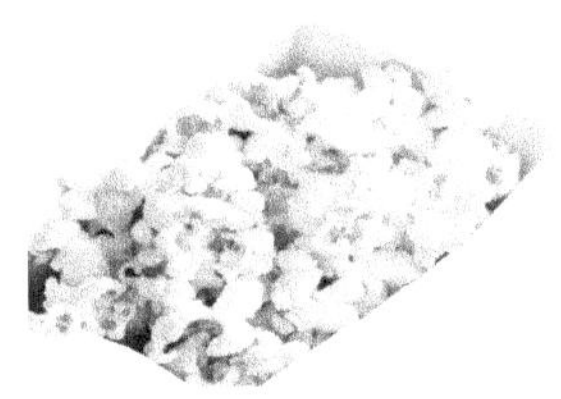

Ingredients:

-A half-cup of popcorn kernels
- Salt

Preparation procedures:

1. Air-pop popcorn as directed by the manufacturer.
2. Move the popcorn to a big bowl when it has popped.
3. Season with salt according to taste.
4. Toss to sprinkle the salt evenly.
5. Present right away.

Duration : 10 minutes
Serving method: Put in a bowl to serve.

Nutritional values: Calories: ~100, Protein: 3g, Carbs: 20g, Fats: 1g, Fibre: 4g

Mixed Nuts

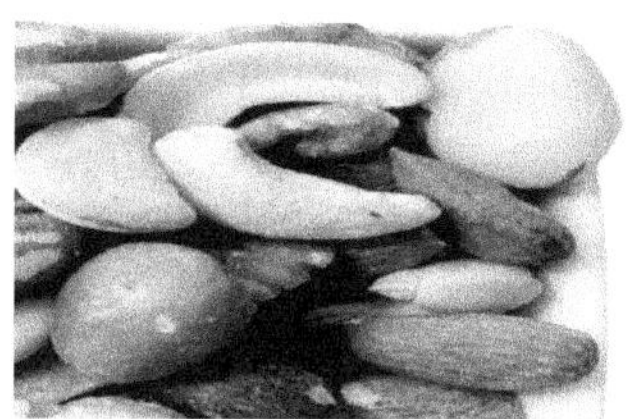

Ingredients:

- ¼ cup unsalted mixed nuts (walnuts, cashews, and almonds)

Preparation procedures:

1. In a small dish, measure out the mixed nuts.
2. For extra taste, you may optionally toast nuts in a dry skillet.
3. If it is burnt, let it cool.
Fourth, as a snack.
5. Keep any leftovers in a well sealed jar.

Duration: 5 minutes
Serving method: This dish should be served in a bowl.

Nutritional values: Calories: ~170, Protein: 5g, Carbs: 6g, Fats: 15g, Fibre: 3g

Cucumber Slices with Greek Yoghourt Dip

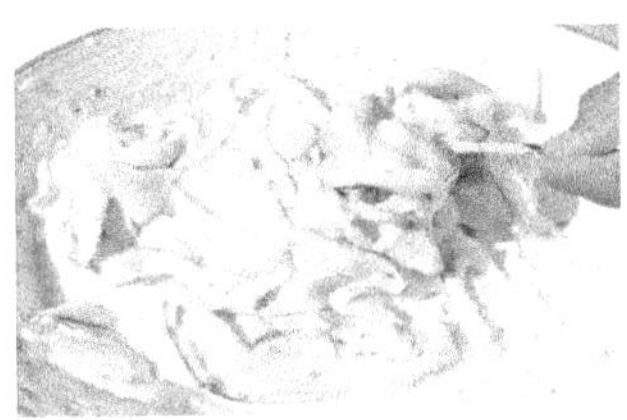

Ingredients:

- 1 medium cucumber, cut into slices
-Half a cup of Greek yoghourt
-One teaspoon of dried herbs, such as dill

Preparation procedures:

1. Combine Greek yoghurt, dried dill, and herbs in a small dish.
2. Cut cucumbers into rounds.
3. Present the yoghurt dip with cucumber slices.
4. Savour as a revitalising snack.
5. Keep any remaining dip refrigerated.

Duration: 5 minutes
Serving method: Present on a platter.

Nutritional values: Calories: ~90, Protein: 5g, Carbs: 8g, Fats: 3g, Fibre: 2g

Desserts

Baked Apples with Cinnamon

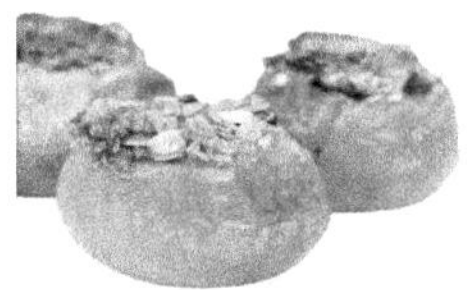

Ingredients:

- two coloured medium apples
- One teaspoon of cinnamon
- One tablespoon of honey (Optional)

Preparation procedure:

1. Set the oven temperature to 175°C (350°F).
2. Put the apples on a baking dish after coreing them.
3. Sprinkle the apples with cinnamon on the interior and outside.
4. If desired, drizzle with honey.
5. Bake until soft, about 20 minutes.

Duration: 25 minutes

Serving method : Warm up in the baking dish.

Nutritional values: Calories: ~100, Protein: 0g, Carbs: 26g, Fats: 0g, Fibre: 4g

Frozen Banana Bites

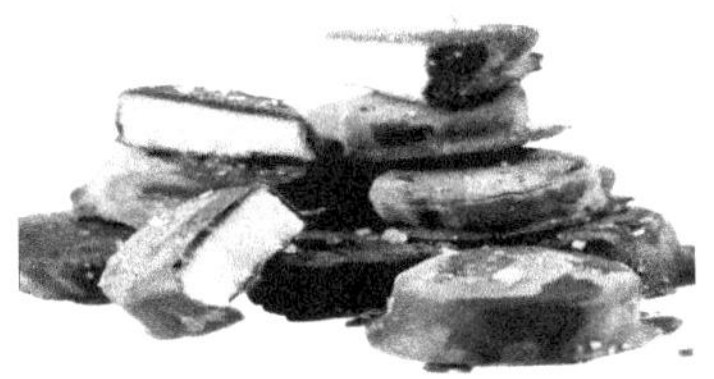

- ½ cup dark chocolate chips
- two medium sliced bananas

Preparation procedures:

1. Use a double boiler or microwave to melt dark chocolate chips.
2. Melt the chocolate and dip each slice of banana in it.
3. Arrange the chocolate-covered slices on a parchment paper-lined baking sheet.
4. To set, freeze for at least an hour.
5. Serve as a dessert when frozen.

Duration: 1 hour (10 minutes for preparation)
Serving method: Present the dish on a platter.

Nutritional values: Calories: ~130, Protein: 1g, Carbs: 24g, Fats: 5g, Fibre: 3g

Berry salad

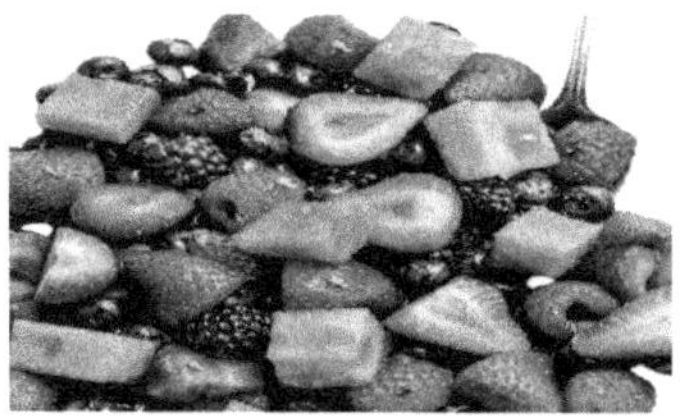

- One cup of cut strawberries
- One cup of blueberries
- One spoonful of honey
- One teaspoon of lemon juice

Preparation procedure:

1. Sliced blueberries and strawberries should be combined in a big basin.
2. Pour lemon juice and honey over it.
3. Gently toss to mix.
4. To improve tastes, let it rest for five minutes.
5. Serve cold.

Duration: **10 minutes**
Serving method: **Transfer to a bowl**

Nutritional values: **Calories: ~90, Protein: 1g, Carbs: 22g, Fats: 0g, Fibre: 5g**

Yoghourt with honey and Walnuts

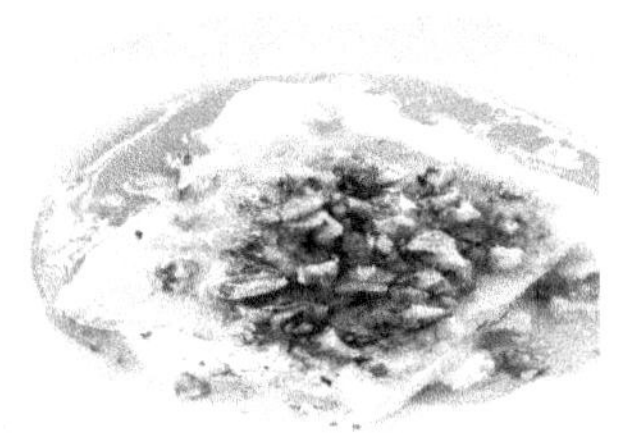

Ingredients:

- 1 cup Greek yoghourt
- Two teaspoons of honey
- 1/4 cup chopped walnuts
- mint leaves to decorate (Optional)

Preparation procedure:

1. Put the Greek yoghurt in a bowl.
2. Pour honey on top of the yoghurt.
3. On top, scatter chopped walnuts.
4. If desired, stir lightly.
5. Serve right away.

Duration: 5 minutes
Serving method: Transfer to a bowl.

Nutritional values: Calories: ~200, Protein: 10g, Carbs: 20g, Fats: 10g, Fibre: 2g

Chocolate Avocado Mousse

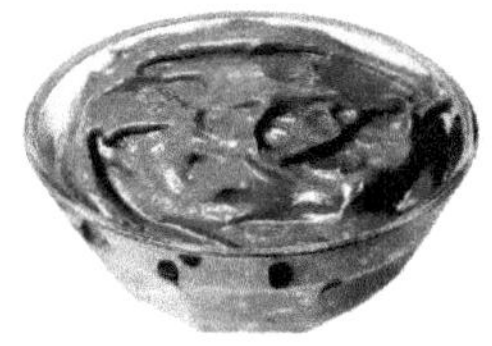

Ingredients:

- 1 ripe Avocado
- Half a cup of cocoa powder
- Half a cup of maple syrup or honey
- One teaspoon of vanilla extract

Preparation procedures:

1. Put the avocado, cocoa powder, honey, and vanilla essence in a food processor or blender.
2. Blend till creamy and smooth.
3. If needed, adjust the sweetness by tasting it.
4. Transfer the mousse to serving plates using a spoon.
5. Before serving, let it cool in the refrigerator for fifteen minutes.

Duration: 20 minutes
Serving method: Present in separate glasses.

Nutritional values: Calories: ~150, Protein: 2g, Carbs: 16g, Fats: 10g, Fibre: 5g

Macaroons with coconut

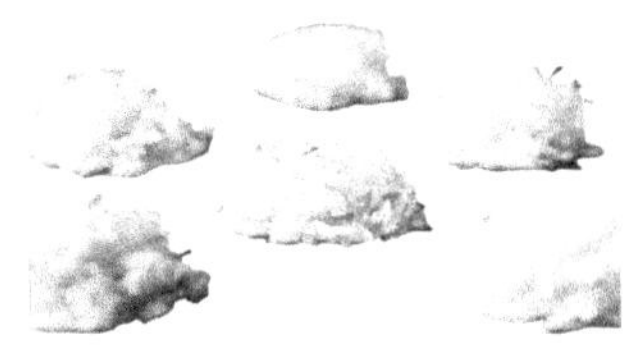

- two cups of unsweetened coconut shreds
- ½ cup condensed milk that has been sweetened
- One teaspoon of vanilla extract
- A pinch of salt

Preparation procedures:

1. Set the oven temperature to 325°F, or 165°C.
2. Combine the salt, vanilla essence, sweetened condensed milk, and shredded coconut in a bowl.
3. Transfer tablespoon-sized portions onto a parchment paper-lined baking sheet.
4. Bake for 15 to 20 minutes, or until it turns golden brown.
5. Before serving, let it cool.

Duration: 25 minutes
Serving method: Present on a dish.

Nutritional values: Calories: ~180, Protein: 2g, Carbs: 16g, Fats: 13g, Fibre: 3g

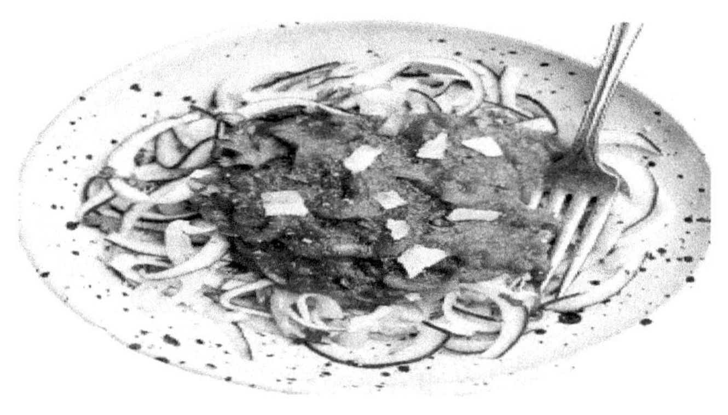

Chapter 4: Staying on Track Lifestyles

Importance of Physical Exercise

Exercise is crucial for gout management, particularly when paired with a well-balanced, gout-friendly diet like the dishes mentioned above. Maintaining a healthy weight, enhancing blood circulation, supporting joint health, and elevating your mood are all benefits of exercise that can lessen gout symptoms and avoid excruciating flare-ups.

The ability to maintain a healthy weight is one of the primary benefits of exercise. Your joints may be further strained by carrying excess weight, especially in gout-prone regions like the knees, ankles, and feet. You may strive toward or maintain a healthy weight by including regular physical exercise, which lessens the strain on these joints and decreases your risk of inflammation. Exercise and nutrient-dense, low-purine foods work together to help you efficiently control your weight and uric acid levels.

Additionally, exercise is essential for maintaining healthy circulation. When uric acid crystals accumulate in your joints, it causes gout, which is characterised by discomfort and inflammation. Your body processes and eliminates excess uric acid more effectively when you exercise because it improves blood flow. Exercises that improve circulation, such as swimming, cycling, and brisk walking, may help your body maintain healthy uric acid levels. Including exercise in your diet after consuming a purine-free diet helps your body eliminate extra uric acid and keep it from building up in your joints.

Exercise not only improves circulation but also fortifies the muscles around your joints. Stronger muscles relieve part of the strain on your joints, which lowers the likelihood of discomfort and inflammation. Strength training with small weights or low-impact activities like yoga or pilates may be especially beneficial for developing muscle around delicate joints without putting undue strain on them. Strengthening activities provide those joints additional support after consuming foods high in antioxidants, vitamins, and minerals that support joint health, allowing for smoother movement and less discomfort.

There are mental and emotional advantages to physical exercise as well. It might be annoying to have gout, particularly when you have to control your discomfort and change your way of life. Endorphins are natural mood enhancers released throughout exercise that make you feel happier, more energetic, and more driven. Maintaining your gout-friendly lifestyle and good eating habits may be made simpler with this mood boost. Additionally, exercise enhances the quality of sleep, which is essential for controlling stress and inflammation. Healthy eating, regular exercise, and sound sleep all contribute to a comprehensive strategy for gout management.

To prevent overstraining, it's critical to select exercises that are easy on your joints. Low-impact exercises like walking, swimming, or cycling might be a good place to start if you're new to exercising or have joint pain. These choices provide cardiovascular advantages that enhance circulation and heart health without being too taxing on the joints.

Physical activity is essential for lowering gout symptoms and enhancing general health because it helps you maintain a healthy weight, increase circulation, build muscle, and elevate your mood. You're taking another step in the right direction toward managing your gout and leading a more active, healthy life by incorporating exercise into your daily routine.

Quality Sleep and Its Impact

Getting enough sleep is crucial for gout management, particularly if you're on a gout-friendly diet like the one mentioned above. You may better control the symptoms of gout by getting enough sleep, which also helps your body heal, lower inflammation, and maintain stable uric acid levels.

Your body has more time to heal and rebuild itself when you get enough sleep. This involves maintaining inflammation and hormone balance, both of which are essential for gout management. Your body may produce more stress hormones if you don't get enough sleep, which might exacerbate gout symptoms by raising inflammation. Consuming meals high in nutrients provides your body with vitamins, minerals, and antioxidants that assist these natural healing processes and may even improve your quality of sleep.

Sleep is crucial for controlling uric acid levels as well. Your kidneys can more effectively filter and eliminate uric acid from your circulation while you're sleeping. This process may be hampered by inadequate sleep, which can result in a buildup of uric acid and potentially cause a flare-up of gout. Low-purine diets and restful sleep work together to help your body better digest and get rid of uric acid, which lowers the chance of excruciating episodes.

Sleep also aids in appetite regulation, preventing cravings for sweet or high-purine meals that might aggravate gout. This plan's meals are rich in fibre, lean proteins, and healthy fats, which will help you feel full and sleep soundly without worrying about hunger in the middle of the night.

To put it simply, getting enough sleep helps your body heal naturally, lower inflammation, and control uric acid levels, all of which improve a gout-friendly diet. When combined, a healthy diet and enough sleep may significantly improve your ability to control gout and feel your best.

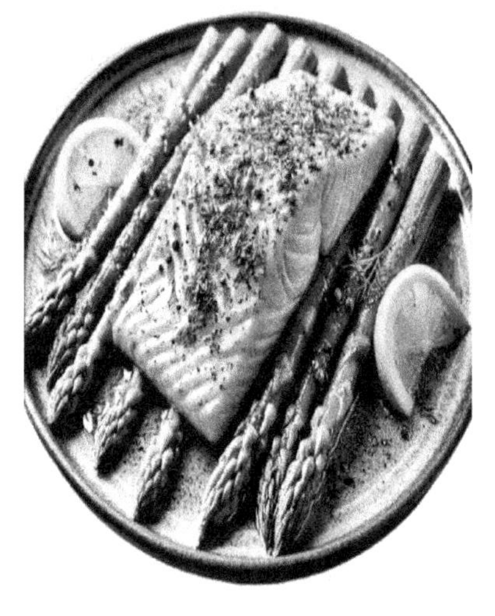

Chapter 5: Conclusion

Congratulations for finishing *The Healthy Gout Diet Recipes for Beginners 2024* You've made a crucial step toward gout management and diet-based health improvement with this book. You now know more about how dietary decisions might affect your body's uric acid levels, resulting in fewer flare-ups and an improved quality of life. Let's go over some of the most crucial lessons you learned along the way.

You studied the fundamentals of gout and its progression in the first few chapters. A kind of arthritis known as gout is brought on by an accumulation of uric acid in the blood, which crystallises in the joints and causes excruciating pain and inflammation. Because certain foods may increase uric acid levels while others can lower them, diet is important in the management of gout. You now know which foods to consume more of, such as vegetables, whole grains, and low-fat dairy, and which to avoid or limit, like alcohol, seafood, red meats, and high-sugar drinks. Having this fundamental understanding is essential to make health-related decisions.

Building a gout-friendly diet is one of the book's primary goals, and you've seen firsthand how to arrange your daily meals for balance and diversity with the help of the organised 14-day meal plan. With a variety of breakfast, lunch, dinner, and snack choices, this meal plan demonstrates that eating a gout-friendly diet doesn't have to mean compromising on taste or pleasure. To maintain a fulfilling and healthful diet, you may keep using and modifying these concepts to develop meal plans that fit your preferences, way of life, and dietary requirements.

One of this guide's most useful sections is the recipe section, which aims to make cooking at home simple and pleasurable. You now have 30 simple, fast recipes at your disposal. Each of the six breakfast, lunch, dinner, snack, and dessert dishes gives you a variety of gout-friendly meals that you can include into your daily routine. You may still enjoy delicious meals while avoiding many of the bad alternatives that might cause gout by learning to create these recipes.

This book has given you vital advice for sustained success in addition to recipes and meals. These pointers assist you in making wise decisions in a variety of dining scenarios, such as cooking for a family, dining out, or attending parties. You now know basic techniques for meal planning, recipe modification, and ingredient substitution that can help you maintain long-term, sustainable diet management.

You have also seen throughout this book how a comprehensive approach to gout care may include regular exercise and the importance of Sleep. You may further lower the likelihood of flare-ups by implementing these lifestyle changes, which provide your body a balanced, healthy environment. This book encourages you to see managing your gout as a way of life that promotes your general well-being in addition to your physical health.

Ultimately, *The Healthy Gout Diet Recipes for Beginners 2024* provides you with the information, resources, and encouragement you need to successfully manage gout and lead a satisfying life free from continual dietary concerns. You have a firm grasp of how nutrition and gout are related, as well as the useful abilities to implement long-lasting, beneficial adjustments. Keep in mind that gout management is a process rather than a fast cure, and that you have the tools at your disposal to help you along the way.

Keep trying out new dishes, consuming a variety of foods, and enjoying your meals. Even if there are obstacles on the way to improved health, merely finishing this book has already allowed you to make amazing strides. You have everything you need to manage your gout, and eventually your efforts will result in better health, less pain, and a stronger feeling of control over your health.

Take what you've learned, continue to follow these routines, and enjoy the process of becoming a healthy version of yourself. Now that you have a lifestyle that suits you, you are ready to succeed.

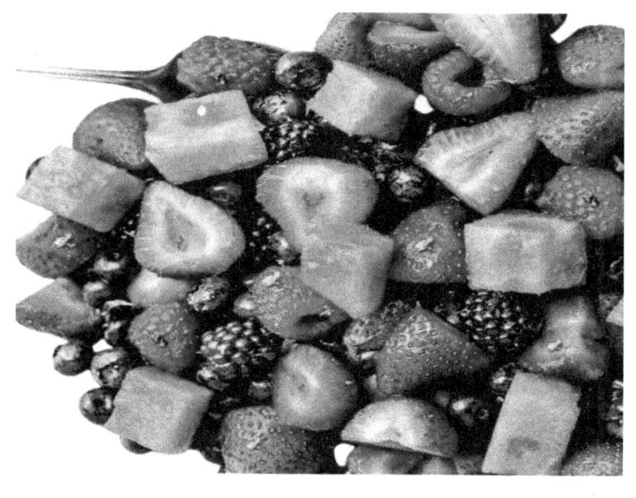

Bonuses

Bonuses

14 days meal plan

Day 1

Almond milk oatmeal with fresh berries and a few walnuts on top

Grilled chicken salad with mixed greens, cucumbers, cherry tomatoes, and olive oil dressing

caramel sticks and apple slices with peanut butter

Baked salmon with quinoa and steamed broccoli

Day 2

Aca and poached egg on whole grain toast with a side of orange slices

Mixed greens salad and lentil soup with whole grain crackers

Celery sticks with hummus and a handful of almonds

Grilled turkey breast with sweet potatoes and steamed spinach

Day 3

Greek yoghourt with chia seeds, topped with sliced strawberries and honey

Wrap with turkey and avocado (whole wheat tortilla), accompanied by baby carrots

Fresh or dried cherries, cucumber slices with hummus

Stir-fried tofu with brown rice, zucchini, and bell peppers

Day 4

Smoothie with banana, spinach, almond milk, and chia seeds

Grilled chicken wrap with spinach, lettuce, and cucumber

Hard-boiled egg, handful of mixed nuts

Baked cod with mashed sweet potatoes and roasted Brussels sprouts

Day 5

Whole grain toast with scrambled eggs and sautéed spinach

Quinoa salad with cucumber, tomato, chickpeas, and feta cheese

Apple slices and low-fat cheese with wheat crackers

Turkey chilli with kidney beans and steamed green beans

Day 6

Whole wheat pancakes with avocado and fresh blueberries on the side

Whole wheat tortilla wrap with spinach and feta

A handful of walnuts and orange slices

Grilled shrimp with couscous and roasted veggies

Day 7

Greek yoghourts parfait with granola, almonds, and mixed berries

Tuna salad in whole grain bread with celery and low-fat mayo accompanied by cucumber slices

Baby carrots with hummus, a banana

Baked chicken breast with roasted butternut squash and asparagus

Day 8

Almond milk, spinach, banana, and blueberries smoothie

Chicken Caesar salad (no croutons) on the grill with steamed broccoli

Cherry tomatoes with low-fat cheese, a handful of mixed nuts

Baked salmon with quinoa and sautéed kale

Day 9

Toast with banana slices, flaxseeds, and almond butter on top

Whole wheat bread turkey sandwich with avocado and lettuce

A handful of cherries and celery sticks with almond butter.

Brown rice, stir-fried veggies, and grilled shrimp

Whole wheat toast and scrambled eggs with sautéed mushrooms

Quinoa bowl with roasted chickpeas, mixed greens, and lemon-tahini dressing

Low-fat yoghurts with berries and apple slices

Grilled cod served with crispy sweet potatoes and steamed broccoli

Greek yoghourt with chia seeds, garnished with mixed berries and honey

Zucchini Noodles with Tomato and Basil

A handful of walnuts and carrot sticks
Dinner: Grilled Shrimp with Steamed Green Beans

Almond milk, banana, spinach, and chia seeds smoothie

Whole wheat crackers and lentil soup with a side salad

Hard-boiled egg and sliced cucumbers

Baked chicken with quinoa and roasted Brussels sprouts

Day 13

avocado and poached egg on whole wheat toast with fresh orange slices on the side

spinach salad with grilled chicken, cherry tomatoes, and olive oil dressing

Apple slices with peanut butter and a handful of almonds

grilled salmon served with brown rice and steamed asparagus

Day 14

Greek yoghourts parfait with mixed berries and granola

Whole wheat tortilla with turkey, avocado wrap and baby carrots on the side

A handful of cherries, cucumber slices with hummus

Stir-fried tofu with brown rice, broccoli, and zucchini

2 weeks Meal planner

Weekly meal *planner*

WEEK: 1

			GROCERY LIST
MONDAY	BREAKFAST		◇
	LUNCH		◇
	DINNER		◇
TUESDAY	BREAKFAST		◇
	LUNCH		◇
	DINNER		◇
WEDNESDAY	BREAKFAST		◇
	LUNCH		◇
	DINNER		◇
THURSDAY	BREAKFAST		◇
	LUNCH		
	DINNER		
FRIDAY	BREAKFAST		SNACKS
	LUNCH		
	DINNER		
SATURDAY	BREAKFAST		
	LUNCH		NOTES
	DINNER		
SUNDAY	BREAKFAST		
	LUNCH		
	DINNER		

Weekly meal *planner*

WEEK: 2

		GROCERY LIST
MONDAY	BREAKFAST	◇
	LUNCH	◇
	DINNER	◇
TUESDAY	BREAKFAST	◇
	LUNCH	◇
	DINNER	◇
WEDNESDAY	BREAKFAST	◇
	LUNCH	◇
	DINNER	◇
THURSDAY	BREAKFAST	◇
	LUNCH	
	DINNER	
FRIDAY	BREAKFAST	SNACKS
	LUNCH	
	DINNER	
SATURDAY	BREAKFAST	
	LUNCH	NOTES
	DINNER	
SUNDAY	BREAKFAST	
	LUNCH	
	DINNER